Scalloped Potatoes

If you want to make an even richer dish, substitute 150 ml/¼ pt of the milk with the same measure of double cream.

Serves 8

900 g/2 lb floury potatoes, peeled and sliced (5 mm/¼ in)
½ onion, thinly sliced
salt and freshly ground black pepper, to taste
40 g/1½ oz butter or margarine
3 tbsp finely chopped onion
25 g/1 oz flour
450 ml/¾ pint semi-skimmed milk
freshly grated nutmeg, to taste

Layer half the potatoes and sliced onion in the slow cooker. Sprinkle lightly with salt and pepper. Melt the butter or margarine in a small pan. Add the chopped onion and flour and cook for 1–2 minutes. Gradually whisk in the milk. Heat to boiling, stirring until thickened, 2–3 minutes. Season the sauce with salt and pepper to taste. Pour half the sauce over the potatoes. Repeat the layers. Cover and cook on High until the potatoes are tender, about 3½ hours. Sprinkle with nutmeg.

Creamy Potatoes and Ham

A quick dish to make, using canned soup for lots of flavour without much effort.

Serves 8

750 g/1¾ lb potatoes, scrubbed and cubed

350 g/12 oz smoked ham, cubed

275 g/10 oz cream of mushroom soup

250 ml/8 fl oz semi-skimmed milk

175 g/6 oz Cheddar cheese, grated

¼ tsp pepper

Combine the potatoes and ham in the slow cooker. Mix in the combined remaining ingredients. Cover and cook on Low for 6–7 hours.

Winter Vegetables Baked in Cream

The season's root vegetables, slow cooked in cream, are a delicious treat.

Serves 6

4 small waxy potatoes, sliced

2 parsnips, sliced

2–3 small leeks (white parts only), sliced

1 fennel bulb, sliced

2 garlic cloves, crushed

½ tsp dried thyme

250 ml/8 fl oz vegetable stock

250 ml/8 fl oz single cream

250 ml/8 fl oz soured cream

2 tbsp cornflour

salt and freshly ground black pepper, to taste

Combine all the ingredients, except the soured cream, cornflour, salt and pepper, in the slow cooker. Cover and cook on High until the vegetables are tender, about 5 hours. Stir in the combined soured cream and cornflour, stirring for 2–3 minutes. Season to taste with salt and pepper.

Spinach Bake

Slow cooked and delicious, this humble spinach recipe, flavoured with basil, thyme and nutmeg, makes a great side dish.

Serves 4–6

275 g/10 oz frozen spinach, thawed

1 small onion, coarsely chopped

1 celery stick, thickly sliced

1 garlic clove

2 tbsp olive oil

½ tsp dried basil

½ tsp dried thyme

a pinch of freshly grated nutmeg

salt and freshly ground black pepper, to taste

2 eggs

50 g/2 oz Emmental or Gruyère cheese, grated

oil, for greasing

25 g/1 oz freshly grated Parmesan cheese

Process the spinach, onion, celery, garlic, oil, herbs and nutmeg in a food processor or blender until very finely chopped. Season to taste with salt and pepper. Add the eggs and process until smooth. Stir in the Emmental or Gruyère cheese. Spoon the mixture into a greased 1 litre/1¾ pint soufflé dish and sprinkle with the Parmesan cheese. Put the soufflé dish on a rack in a 5.5 litre/9½ pint slow cooker. Cover and cook on Low until the mixture is set and a sharp knife inserted half-way between the centre and the edge comes out clean, about 4 hours.

Spaghetti Squash Parmesan

The delicate flavour of the squash is complemented by the combination of Italian herb seasoning and Parmesan cheese.

Serves 4

1 spaghetti squash, about 900 g/2 lb
2 spring onions, sliced
1 garlic clove, crushed
1 tbsp butter or margarine
50 ml/2 fl oz vegetable stock
1½ tsp dried Italian herb seasoning
50 g/2 oz freshly grated Parmesan cheese
salt and freshly ground black pepper, to taste

Cut about 2.5 cm/1 in off the ends of the squash and put the squash in the slow cooker. Cover and cook on High until just tender, 3–4 hours on High or 6–8 hours on Low. Cut the squash lengthways into halves. Scoop out and discard the seeds. Fluff the strands of squash with the tines of a fork, leaving the squash in the shells.

Sauté the spring onions and garlic in the butter or margarine in a small pan until tender, 3 to 4 minutes. Stir in the stock and Italian herb seasoning and heat to boiling. Spoon half the mixture into each squash half and toss. Sprinkle with Parmesan cheese and season to taste with salt and pepper.

Courgette and Mushroom Soufflé

Serve the soufflé immediately it soars above the dish!

Serves 8

4 eggs

175 ml/6 fl oz full-fat milk

25 g/1 oz plain flour

450 g/1 lb courgettes, finely chopped

100 g/4 oz mushrooms, sliced

2 tbsp snipped fresh chives or chopped parsley

1 garlic clove, crushed

½ tsp dried Italian herb seasoning

¾ tsp salt

a pinch of pepper

50 g/2 oz freshly grated Parmesan cheese

paprika

Beat the eggs, milk and flour in a bowl until smooth. Mix in the remaining ingredients, except 25 g/1 oz of the Parmesan cheese and a little paprika. Pour the mixture into a 1.5 litre/2½ pint soufflé dish or casserole. Sprinkle with the remaining Parmesan cheese and a little paprika. Put the soufflé dish on a rack in a 5.5 litre/9½ pint slow cooker. Cover and cook on High until puffed and set, about 4 hours. Serve immediately.

Courgette and Corn Timbale with Roasted Red Pepper Sauce

A summer treat made with fresh seasonal vegetables and served with a bright red pepper sauce.

Serves 6

4 courgettes, coarsely grated

225 g/8 oz sweetcorn, thawed if frozen

1½ onions, chopped

15 g/½ oz fresh coriander, chopped

50 ml/2 fl oz dry white wine

5 eggs

150 ml/¼ pint evaporated milk

75 g/3 oz Cheddar cheese, grated

½ tsp salt

a pinch of pepper

Roasted Red Pepper Sauce

Combine all the ingredients, except the Roasted Red Pepper Sauce, in a 1 litre/1¾ pint casserole or soufflé dish. Put on a rack in a 5.5 litre/9½ pint slow cooker. Cover and cook on High until the vegetables are tender, about 4 hours. Serve with Roasted Red Pepper Sauce.

Tomato Pudding

Bought croûtons can be substituted for home-made if you want to make this a super-quick dish.

Serves 6

1 celery, finely chopped

1 onion, finely chopped

½ green pepper, finely chopped

400 g/14 oz can chopped tomatoes

½ tsp celery seeds

½ tsp dried marjoram

1 tbsp light brown sugar

salt and freshly ground black pepper, to taste

1 tbsp cornflour

2 tbsp cold water

Crispy Croûtons

Combine all the ingredients, except the salt, pepper, cornflour, water and Crispy Croûtons, in the slow cooker. Season to taste with salt and pepper. Cover and cook on High for 2 hours. Stir in the combined cornflour and water, stirring for 2–3 minutes. Stir in the Crispy Croûtons. Cover and cook on High 15 for minutes.

Tomato Sauce

You can't beat a home-made fresh tomato sauce to add flavour to dishes, or to serve with pasta and Parmesan or Mozzarella cheese for a simple meal. This sauce tastes particularly good made with tomatoes when in season, as these will have the most sweetness. You can also make the sauce using 2½ cans of chopped plum tomatoes. The sauce is ideal for freezing in batches so that you can add it to slow-cooker recipes instead of using a ready-made sauce from a jar. Remember to thaw it completely, and preferably allow it to reach room temperature before adding it to the slow cooker.

Serves 6

1 kg/2¼ lb tomatoes peeled, seeded and chopped

1 onion, chopped

1 garlic clove, crushed

120 ml/4 fl oz olive oil

2 tsp dried oregano

2 tsp dried basil

2 tsp cayenne pepper

2 tsp salt

2 tsp freshly ground black pepper

½ tsp cinnamon

Put the tomatoes, onion, garlic and olive oil in the slow cooker. Stir in the oregano, basil, cayenne pepper, salt, pepper and cinnamon. Cover and cook on Low for 10–15 hours.

Spinach and Cheese Noodle Pudding

This is popular with all the family, so be forewarned – everyone will
want seconds!

Serves 8

225 g/8 oz cottage cheese

75 g/3 oz soft cheese, at room temperature

3 large eggs, lightly beaten

300 ml/½ pint full-fat milk

75 g/3 oz raisins

½ tsp ground cinnamon

275 g/10 oz frozen spinach, thawed

100 g/4 oz egg noodles, cooked al dente

½ tsp salt

freshly grated Parmesan cheese

paprika, to garnish

Combine the cottage cheese and soft cheese. Mix in the eggs, blending well. Mix in the remaining ingredients, except the Parmesan cheese and paprika. Spoon into a 1 litre/1¾ pint soufflé dish or casserole and sprinkle with the Parmesan cheese and a little paprika. Put the soufflé dish on a rack in a 5.5 litre/9½ pint slow cooker. Cover and cook on Low until set, about 4 hours.

Note: this recipe can also be cooked in a 2.75 litre/4¾ pint slow cooker, without using a soufflé dish. The cooking time will be about 3½ hours.

Hungarian Noodle Pudding

This kugel, flavoured with raspberry preserve and almonds, can also be served as a dessert!

Serves 10

4 eggs, separated

100 g/4 oz caster sugar

250 ml/8 fl oz soured cream

1 tbsp grated orange zest

2 tsp ground cinnamon

oil, for greasing

225 g/8 oz egg noodles or small elbow macaroni, cooked

2 tbsp butter or margarine

175 g/6 oz seedless raspberry preserve, melted

50 g/2 oz almonds, chopped

Beat the egg yolks and sugar in a small bowl until thick and lemon-coloured, about 5 minutes. Beat in the soured cream, orange zest and cinnamon. Beat the egg whites in a large clean bowl with clean beaters until stiff peaks form. Fold the yolk mixture into the egg whites. Grease the inside of the slow cooker.

Mix the noodles or macaroni, butter or margarine and egg mixture in a large bowl. Spoon half the mixture into the greased slow cooker. Spoon the preserve over the noodles and sprinkle with half the almonds. Top with the remaining noodle mixture and the remaining almonds. Cover and cook on High until set, about 1 hour. Serve from the slow cooker or invert on to a serving platter.

Cherry and Peach Dessert Kugel

The kugel is a staple of Jewish cuisine; the word itself is Yiddish for 'ball' and refers to the fact that the noodles were often shaped into a ball enclosing the sweet or salty filling.

Serves 10

4 eggs, separated

100 g/4 oz caster sugar

250 ml/8 fl oz soured cream

1 tbsp grated orange zest

2 tsp ground cinnamon

oil, for greasing

225 g/8 oz egg noodles or small elbow macaroni, cooked

2 tbsp butter or margarine

225 g/8 oz cottage cheese

225 g/8 oz canned peaches, drained and chopped

50 g/2 oz dried cherries

50 g/2 oz almonds, chopped

Beat the egg yolks and sugar in a small bowl until thick and lemon-coloured, about 5 minutes. Beat in the soured cream, orange zest and cinnamon. Beat the egg whites in a large clean bowl with clean beaters, until stiff peaks form. Fold the yolk mixture into the egg whites. Grease the inside of the slow cooker.

Mix the noodles or macaroni, butter or margarine, cheese, peaches, cherries and egg mixture in a large bowl. Spoon half the mixture into the greased slow cooker and sprinkle with half the almonds. Top with the remaining noodle mixture and the remaining almonds. Cover and cook on High until set, about 1 hour. Serve from the slow cooker or invert on to a serving platter.

Mushroom Bread Pudding

This can be cooked after assembling, but is more flavourful if refrigerated overnight.

Serves 8

225 g/8 oz Italian or sourdough bread, cubed (2.5 cm/1 in)

olive oil cooking spray

1 tsp dried thyme

225 g/8 oz brown cap mushrooms, thinly sliced

1 celery stick, thinly sliced

2 small onions, thinly sliced

¾ green pepper, thinly sliced

1 garlic clove, crushed

1–2 tbsp olive oil, plus extra for greasing

250 ml/8 fl oz single cream

250 ml/8 fl oz full-fat milk

4 eggs, lightly beaten

½ tsp salt

a pinch of pepper

25 g/1 oz Parmesan cheese, finely grated

Spray the bread cubes lightly with cooking spray. Sprinkle with the thyme and toss. Bake on a baking sheet at 190ºC/gas 5/fan oven 170ºC until just beginning to brown, about 15 minutes. Sauté the mushrooms, celery, onions, pepper and garlic in the oil in a large frying pan until tender, about 8 minutes. Grease the inside of the slow cooker.

Mix the cream, milk, eggs, salt and pepper until well blended in a large bowl. Mix in the bread cubes and sautéed vegetables. Spoon into the slow cooker pot and sprinkle with the Parmesan. Refrigerate overnight. Put the crock in the slow cooker. Cover and cook on High until set, 4½ to 5 hours.

Note: the bread pudding can also be cooked in a greased 1.5 litre/2½ pint soufflé dish or casserole. Put on a rack in a 5.5 litre/9½ pint slow cooker. Cover and cook on High for 5 hours.

Savoury Oatmeal

This is the perfect side dish for any meat, poultry or fish entrée.

Serves 6

100 g/4 oz pinhead oatmeal

900 ml/1½ pints vegetable stock

250 ml/8 fl oz dry white wine

175 g/6 oz small chestnut mushrooms, sliced

1 leek (white part only), halved and thinly sliced

1 garlic clove, crushed

1 tsp dried basil

1 tsp dried oregano

1 tsp dried thyme

1 tsp salt

1 tsp pepper

50–75 g/2–3 oz freshly grated Parmesan cheese

Combine all the ingredients, except the cheese, in the slow cooker. Cover and cook on Low for 6–8 hours. Stir in the cheese.

Polenta

Creamy polenta is a wonderful side dish, and this basic recipe has many possible variations.

Serves 6

75 g/3 oz yellow polenta
450 ml/¾ pint water
2 tbsp butter or margarine
50 g/2 oz freshly grated Parmesan cheese
salt and freshly ground black pepper, to taste

Mix the polenta and water in the slow cooker. Cover and cook on High for 1½ hours, stirring once after 45 minutes. Stir in the butter or margarine and cheese. Cover and cook for 15 minutes (polenta should be soft, but should hold its shape). Season to taste with salt and pepper.

Blue Cheese Polenta

There are many varieties of crumbly blue cheese to choose from and all should work well.

Serves 6

75 g/3 oz yellow polenta
450 ml/¾ pint water
2 tbsp butter or margarine
50 g/2 oz blue cheese, crumbled
salt and freshly ground black pepper, to taste

Mix the polenta and water in the slow cooker. Cover and cook on High for 1½ hours, stirring once after 45 minutes. Stir in the butter or margarine and cheese. Cover and cook for 15 minutes (polenta should be soft, but should hold its shape). Season to taste with salt and pepper.

Goats' Cheese Polenta

Goats' cheese has a characteristic, delicious tartness. Recent studies have shown that it is higher in protein than cheese made from cow's milk.

Serves 6

75 g/3 oz yellow polenta
450 ml/¾ pint water
2 tbsp butter or margarine
25–50 g/1–2 oz goats' cheese, crumbled
salt and freshly ground black pepper, to taste

Mix the polenta and water in the slow cooker. Cover and cook on High for 1½ hours, stirring once after 45 minutes. Stir in the butter or margarine and cheese. Cover and cook for 15 minutes (polenta should be soft, but should hold its shape). Season to taste with salt and pepper.

Garlic Polenta

You could sauté the garlic mixture while the polenta is cooking

instead of beforehand.

Serves 6

½ onion, finely chopped

4–6 garlic cloves, crushed

1 tbsp olive oil

75 g/3 oz yellow polenta

450 ml/¾ pint water

2 tbsp butter or margarine

salt and freshly ground black pepper

Sauté the onion and garlic in the olive oil in a small frying pan until tender, 2–3 minutes. Mix the polenta and water in the slow cooker. Cover and cook on High for 45 minutes. Stir, re-cover and cook for a further 30 minutes. Add the onion and garlic mixture, re-cover and cook for a further 15 minutes. Stir in the butter or margarine, re-cover and cook for 15 minutes (polenta should be soft, but should hold its shape). Season to taste with salt and pepper.

Roasted Pepper and Goats' Cheese Polenta

Sweet red pepper perfectly complements the slight sharpness of goats' cheese.

Serves 6

75 g/3 oz yellow polenta

450 ml/¾ pint water

2 tbsp butter or margarine

50–100 g/2–4 oz goats' cheese, crumbled

½ roasted red pepper, chopped

salt and freshly ground black pepper

Mix the polenta and water in the slow cooker. Cover and cook on High for 1½ hours, stirring once after 45 minutes. Stir in the butter or margarine, cheese and chopped pepper. Cover and cook for 15 minutes (polenta should be soft, but should hold its shape). Season to taste with salt and pepper.

Basil Polenta

To my mind basil is the Italian herb. You can buy it growing in small pots in supermarkets and it's a great herb to keep on the windowsill for countless recipes.

Serves 6

3 spring onions, sliced

2 garlic cloves, crushed

1 tsp dried basil

2 tsp olive oil

75 g/3 oz yellow polenta

450 ml/¾ pint water

2 tbsp butter or margarine

50 g/2 oz freshly grated Parmesan cheese

salt and freshly ground black pepper, to taste

Sauté the spring onions, garlic and basil in the olive oil in a large pan until tender, about 2 minutes. Mix the polenta and water in the slow cooker. Cover and cook on High for 45 minutes. Stir, re-cover and cook for a further 30 minutes. Add the the onion mixture, re-cover and cook for a further 15 minutes. Stir in the butter or margarine, re-cover and cook for 15 minutes (polenta should be soft, but should hold its shape). Season to taste with salt and pepper.

Cheese and Rice Torta

Spinach, cherry tomatoes, olives and Mozzarella flavour this unique rice dish.

Serves 6

225 g/8 oz arborio rice, cooked until al dente
275 g/10 oz frozen spinach, thawed and squeezed dry
2 eggs, lightly beaten
1 onion, finely chopped
65 g/2½ oz cherry tomatoes, halved
75 g/3 oz Mozzarella cheese, grated
40 g/1½ oz black olives, sliced
½ tsp salt
a pinch of pepper
oil, for greasing

Combine the rice, spinach and eggs in a bowl. Mix in the remaining ingredients. Spoon into a greased 18 cm/7 in springform cake tin. Put the tin on a rack in a 5.5 litre/9½ pint slow cooker. Cover and cook on Low until set, about 3 hours. Remove the cake tin and cool on a wire rack for 5–10 minutes. Loosen the side of the tin and cut into wedges.

Buttermilk Bread

Yummy with soups and casseroles – serve warm with butter.

Serves 8

175 g/6 oz plain flour

2 tsp baking powder

a pinch of bicarbonate of soda

½ tsp salt

50 g/2 oz cold butter or margarine, cut into pieces

175 ml/6 fl oz buttermilk

1 tbsp dried parsley

oil, for greasing

Combine the flour, baking powder, bicarbonate of soda and salt in a bowl. Cut in the butter until the mixture resembles small crumbs. Stir in the buttermilk and parsley.

Knead the dough on a floured surface for 1–2 minutes. Pat the dough into a greased 18 cm/7 in springform cake tin and put on a rack in a 5.5 litre/9½ pint slow cooker. Cover and cook on High until a cocktail stick inserted into the centre comes out clean, 2–2½ hours. Cool in the tin on a wire rack for 10 minutes. Remove the side of the tin. Break off pieces to serve.

Pepper and Herb Bread

Originally buttermilk was the tartly flavoured liquid left behind after churning butter out of milk but nowadays you can buy cartons of cultured buttermilk from the supermarket.

Serves 8

175 g/6 oz plain flour

2 tsp baking powder

a pinch of bicarbonate of soda

½ tsp salt

50 g/2 oz cold butter or margarine, cut into pieces

175 ml/6 fl oz buttermilk

2 tsp dried chives

1 tsp coarse ground pepper

1 tsp dried dill

oil, for greasing

Combine the flour, baking powder, bicarbonate of soda and salt in a bowl. Cut in the butter until the mixture resembles small crumbs. Stir in the buttermilk, half the chives and all the pepper and dill.

Knead the dough on a floured surface for 1–2 minutes. Pat the dough into a greased 18 cm/7 in springform cake tin and put on a rack in a 5.5 litre/9½ pint slow cooker. Cover and cook on High until a cocktail stick inserted into the centre comes out clean, 2–2½ hours. Cool in the tin on a wire rack for 10 minutes. Sprinkle the top of the bread with the remaining dried chives. Remove the side of the tin. Break off pieces to serve.

Rosemary and Raisin Bread

I have specified dried rosemary but if you are lucky enough to have it growing in your garden you could use 1 tsp of fresh leaves, chopped, instead.

Serves 8

175 g/6 oz plain flour

2 tsp baking powder

a pinch of bicarbonate of soda

½ tsp salt

50 g/2 oz cold butter or margarine, cut into pieces

175 ml/6 fl oz buttermilk

1 tbsp dried parsley

50 g/2 oz sultanas

½ tsp dried, crushed rosemary

oil, for greasing

Combine the flour, baking powder, bicarbonate of soda and salt in a bowl. Cut in the butter or margarine until the mixture resembles small crumbs. Stir in the buttermilk, parsley, sultanas and rosemary.

Knead the dough on a floured surface for 1–2 minutes. Pat the dough into a greased 18 cm/7 in springform cake tin and put on a rack in a 5.5 litre/9½ pint slow cooker. Cover and cook on High until a cocktail stick inserted into the centre comes out clean, 2–2½ hours. Cool in the tin on a wire rack for 10 minutes. Remove the side of the tin. Break off pieces to serve.

Spoon Bread

Use a spoon to serve this bread in shallow bowls topped with casserole, or invert the bread on to a serving plate and break it into pieces.

Serves 6–8

175 ml/6 fl oz boiling water

50 g/2 oz yellow polenta

2 tsp butter or margarine, at room temperature

2 egg yolks

75 ml/2½ fl oz buttermilk

½ tsp salt

½ tsp sugar

½ tsp baking powder

¼ tsp bicarbonate of soda

2 egg whites, whisked to stiff peaks

oil, for greasing

Stir the boiling water into the polenta in a bowl. Leave to cool until barely warm, stirring occasionally. Stir in the butter or margarine and egg yolks, blending well. Mix in the buttermilk and combined remaining ingredients, except the egg whites. Fold in the egg whites.

Pour the batter into a greased 18 cm/ 7 in springform cake tin. Put the tin on a rack in a 5.5 litre/9½ pint slow cooker. Cover and cook on High until a cocktail stick inserted into the centre of the bread comes out clean, 2½–2¾ hours. Serve immediately.

Fruited Bran Bread

Serve this bread warm with honey or jam – fabulous!

Serves 16

175 g/6 oz plain flour

50 g/2 oz wholemeal flour

2 tsp baking powder

½ tsp bicarbonate of soda

½ tsp salt

25 g/1 oz bran flakes

175 ml/2½ fl oz buttermilk

175 g/6 oz light brown sugar

50 g/2 oz butter or margarine, melted

1 egg

175 g/6 oz dried mixed fruit

50 g/2 oz walnuts, chopped

oil, for greasing

Combine the flours, baking powder, bicarbonate of soda, salt and bran flakes in a medium bowl. Add the buttermilk, brown sugar, butter or margarine and egg, mixing until the dry ingredients are just moistened. Gently fold in the dried fruit and walnuts.

Pour the batter into a greased and floured 23 x 13 cm/9 x 5 in loaf tin. Put the tin on a rack in a 5.5 litre/9½ pint slow cooker. Cover and cook on High until a cocktail stick inserted into the centre of the loaf comes out clean, 2–3 hours. Cool in the tin on a wire rack for 5 minutes. Remove from the tin and finish cooling on the wire rack.

Apricot and Date Bran Bread

A tasty and nutritious bread that is moist enough to enjoy on its own but is even better sliced and buttered.

Serves 16

175 g/6 oz plain flour

50 g/2 oz wholemeal flour

2 tsp baking powder

½ tsp bicarbonate of soda

½ tsp salt

25 g/1 oz bran flakes

175 ml/2½ fl oz buttermilk

175 g/6 oz light brown sugar

50 g/2 oz butter or margarine, melted

1 egg

40 g/1½ oz dates, chopped

40 g/1½ oz dried apricots, chopped

50 g/2 oz pecan nuts, chopped

oil, for greasing

Combine the flours, baking powder, bicarbonate of soda, salt and bran flakes in a medium bowl. Add the buttermilk, brown sugar, butter or margarine and egg, mixing until the dry ingredients are just moistened. Gently fold in the dates, apricots and nuts.

Pour the batter into a greased and floured 23 x 13 cm/9 x 5 in loaf tin. Put the tin on a rack in a 5.5 litre/9½ pint slow cooker. Cover and cook on High until a cocktail stick inserted into the centre of the loaf comes out clean, 2–3 hours. Cool in the tin on a wire rack for 5 minutes. Remove from the tin and finish cooling on the wire rack.

Pumpkin and Pecan Bread

Next time you cook some pumpkin or squash, make extra to use in this tasty bread.

Serves 16

225 g/8 oz pumpkin, cooked and mashed

50 g/2 oz butter or margarine, at room temperature

100 g/4 oz caster sugar

100 g/4 oz light brown sugar

120 ml/4 fl oz semi-skimmed milk

2 eggs

225 g/8 oz plain flour

2 tsp baking powder

½ tsp bicarbonate of soda

¾ tsp salt

1½ tsp ground cinnamon

¼–½ tsp ground mace

50 g/2 oz pecan nuts, toasted and chopped

oil, for greasing

Beat the pumpkin, butter or margarine and sugars in a bowl until well blended. Mix in the milk and eggs. Mix in the combined dry ingredients. Mix in the pecan nuts.

Spoon the batter into a greased 23 x 13 cm/ 9 x 5 in loaf tin and put on a rack in a 5.5 litre/9½ pint slow cooker. Cover and cook on

High until a cocktail stick inserted into the centre of the bread comes out clean, about 3½ hours. Cool in the tin on a wire rack for 5 minutes. Remove from the tin and finish cooling on the wire rack.

Brown Sugar Banana Bread

Apple sauce adds moistness to this banana bread with its caramel flavour from the brown sugar. Make your own apple sauce if you have time by cooking 1 peeled, cored and sliced cooking apple in a small pan with 1 tbsp water until very soft.

Serves 16

50 g/2 oz butter or margarine, at room temperature

50 ml/2 fl oz ready-made apple sauce

2 eggs

2 tbsp semi-skimmed milk or water

175 g/6 oz light brown sugar

3 ripe bananas, mashed

200 g/7 oz plain flour

2 tsp baking powder

½ tsp bicarbonate of soda

¼ tsp salt

25 g/1 oz walnuts or pecan nuts, coarsely chopped

oil, for greasing

Beat the butter or margarine, apple sauce, eggs, milk and brown sugar in a large bowl until smooth. Add the bananas and mix at low speed. Beat at high speed for 1–2 minutes. Mix in the combined flour, baking powder, bicarbonate of soda and salt. Mix in the walnuts or pecan nuts.

Pour the batter into a greased 23 x 13 cm/ 9 x 5 in loaf tin. Put the tin on a rack in a 5.5 litre/9½ pint slow cooker. Cover and cook on High until a cocktail stick inserted into the centre of the bread comes out clean, 2–3 hours. Cool in the tin on a wire rack for 5 minutes. Remove the bread from the tin and finish cooling on the wire rack.

Apple and Pecan Nut Banana Bread

You can ring the changes with this tasty bread and use any dried fruit or nut you prefer.

Serves 12

6 tbsp butter or margarine, at room temperature

100 g/4 oz caster sugar

2 eggs

3 ripe bananas, mashed

200 g/7 oz self-raising flour

½ tsp salt

10 g/¼oz dried apples, chopped

50 g/2 oz pecan nuts, chopped

oil, for greasing

Beat the butter or margarine and sugar in a large bowl until fluffy. Beat in the eggs and bananas. Mix in the flour and salt. Mix in the dried apples and pecan nuts.

Pour the batter into a greased 23 x 13 cm/ 9 x 5 in loaf tin. Put on a rack in a 5.5 litre/9½ pint slow cooker. Cover and cook on High until a wooden skewer inserted into the centre of the bread comes out clean, about 3½ hours. Cool on a wire rack for 5 minutes. Remove from the tin and finish cooling on the wire rack.

Boston Brown Bread

The dough for this moist polenta, walnut and raisin bread is steamed
in two tins in the slow cooker.

MAKES 2 Loaves, each serves 6–8

65 g/2½ oz wholemeal flour
50 g/2 oz yellow polenta
40 g/1½ oz walnuts, chopped
50 g/2 oz raisins
2 tbsp light brown sugar
¾ tsp bicarbonate of soda
½ tsp salt
150 ml/¼ pint semi-skimmed milk
75 g/3 oz golden syrup
1 tbsp lemon juice
oil, for greasing

Combine all the ingredients, except the milk, golden syrup and lemon juice, in a bowl. Add the combined milk, golden syrup and lemon juice, mixing well. Spoon the mixture into two greased and floured 450 g/1 lb tins. Cover the tops of the tins with greased foil, securing it with string.

Stand the tins in the slow cooker. Add enough boiling water to come half-way up the sides of the tins, making sure the foil does not touch the water. Cover and cook on High for 2 hours. Turn the heat to Low and cook until a wooden skewer inserted into the breads comes out clean, about 4 hours. Uncover the tins and stand on a wire rack to cool for 10 minutes. Loosen the sides of the bread by gently rolling the tins on the worktop, or remove the bases of the tins and push the breads through.

Roasted Chilli Cornbread

This cornbread is extra moist and chilli hot! Reduce the amount of chilli if you prefer it a bit milder.

Serves 8

¼ small red pepper, chopped

¼ poblano or other mild chilli, chopped

¼ jalapeño or other medium-hot chilli, chopped

1 large spring onion, chopped

oil, for greasing

75 g/3 oz plain flour

25 g/1 oz yellow polenta

2 tbsp light brown sugar

1½ tsp baking powder

¼ tsp ground cumin

¼ tsp dried oregano

¼ tsp salt

1 egg, lightly beaten

120 ml/4 fl oz buttermilk

25 g/1 oz sweetcorn

2 tbsp finely chopped fresh coriander

Cook the pepper, chillies and spring onion in a lightly greased frying pan over medium heat until tender, about 5 minutes. Reserve. Combine the flour, polenta, brown sugar, baking powder, cumin, oregano and salt in a medium bowl. Add the combined egg and buttermilk, mixing until just combined. Stir in the sautéed vegetables, sweetcorn and coriander.

Pour the batter into a greased and floured 18 cm/7 in springform cake tin. Put the tin on a rack in a 5.5 litre/9½ pint slow cooker. Cover and cook on High until a cocktail stick inserted into the centre of the bread comes out clean, about 2 hours. Cool in the tin on a wire rack for 10 minutes. Serve warm.

Parmesan Bread

This melty cheese bread is a perfect accompaniment to soups and casseroles. Choose an oval or round loaf that will fit into your slow cooker.

Serves 6–8

1 small ciabatta loaf
75 g/3 oz butter or margarine, at room temperature
25 g/1 oz freshly grated Parmesan cheese

Without cutting all the way through the base of the loaf, cut the bread into six to eight slices. Spread both sides of the bread slices with the combined butter or margarine and Parmesan cheese. Wrap the loaf securely in foil. Put in the slow cooker and cook on Low for 2 hours.

Note: the bread can also be baked at 180ºC/gas 4/fan oven 160ºC until warm, about 20 minutes.

Brunch Bread Pudding

This bread pudding is assembled in advance and refrigerated overnight before cooking. Make the pudding in a soufflé dish or cook it directly in the crock.

Serves 6

275 g/10 oz stale French bread, cubed (1 cm/½ in)
75 g/3 oz dried apricots, chopped
50 g/2 oz flaked almonds
3 eggs
100 g/4 oz sugar
600 ml/1 pint milk
1 tsp vanilla essence
1 tsp ground cinnamon
warm maple syrup, to serve

Combine the bread cubes, apricots and almonds in a large bowl. Beat the eggs in a large bowl until thick and pale coloured, about 5 minutes. Beat in the sugar, milk, vanilla and cinnamon. Pour over the bread mixture and toss. Spoon into a 1.5 litre/2½ pint soufflé dish or casserole. Refrigerate, covered, overnight.

Put the soufflé dish on a rack in a 5.5 litre/9½ pint slow cooker. Cover and cook on High until the pudding is set, about 5 hours. Serve warm with maple syrup.

Sloppy Joes

A great sandwich for kids of all ages! Serve with lots of pickles and fresh vegetable relishes.

Serves 6–8

450 g/1 lb lean minced beef

oil, for greasing

2 onions, chopped

1 green or red pepper, chopped

2 garlic cloves, crushed

250 ml/8 fl oz tomato ketchup

120 ml/4 fl oz water

50 g/2 oz light brown sugar

2 tbsp prepared mustard

2 tsp celery seeds

2 tsp chilli powder

salt and freshly ground black pepper, to taste

6–8 wholemeal burger buns, toasted

sliced cornichons or pickles, fresh relishes, to serve

Cook the minced beef in a lightly greased frying pan until browned, crumbling with a fork. Combine the minced beef and the remaining ingredients, except the salt, pepper and buns, in the slow cooker. Cover and cook on High for 2–3 hours. Season to taste with salt and pepper. Serve in buns with cornichons, pickles and relishes.

Vegetarian Joes

A great meat-free alternative to Sloppy Joes but you don't have to be vegetarian to enjoy it!

Serves 6–8

225 g/8 oz textured vegetable protein

100 g/4 oz mushrooms, sliced

oil, for greasing

2 onions, chopped

1 green or red pepper, chopped

2 garlic cloves, crushed

250 ml/8 fl oz tomato ketchup

375 ml/13 fl oz water

50 g/2 oz light brown sugar

2 tbsp prepared mustard

2 tsp celery seeds

2 tsp chilli powder

salt and freshly ground black pepper, to taste

6–8 wholemeal burger buns, toasted

sliced cornichons or pickles, fresh relishes, to serve

Cook the textured vegetable protein and mushrooms in a lightly greased frying pan until browned, crumbling with a fork. Combine with the remaining ingredients, except the salt, pepper and buns, in the slow cooker. Cover and cook on High for 2–3 hours. Season to taste with salt and pepper. Serve in buns with cornichons, pickles and relishes.

Cheeseburger Joes

Look out for mild American-style hot-dog mustard on supermarket shelves to use in this recipe.

Serves 12

900 g/2 lb lean minced beef

2 small onions, chopped

1 small green pepper, chopped

225 g/8 oz mushrooms, sliced

3 large garlic cloves, crushed

100 g/4 oz bacon, cooked until crisp and crumbled

100 g/4 oz sweet pickle relish

120 ml/4 fl oz yellow mustard

175 ml/6 fl oz tomato ketchup

1 tbsp Worcestershire sauce

225 g/8 oz processed cheese, cubed

salt and freshly ground black pepper, to taste

12 burger buns, toasted

Cook the beef, onion and pepper over medium heat in a large frying pan until the beef is browned, crumbling it with a fork. Transfer to the slow cooker. Add the remaining ingredients, except the salt, pepper and buns. Cover and cook on Low for 2–3 hours. Season to taste with salt and pepper. Serve on buns.

Vino Joes

This grown-up version of the family favourite, Sloppy Joes, is flavoured with red wine, Worcestershire sauce and Dijon mustard.

Serves 12

450 g/1 lb lean minced beef

2 small onions, chopped

1 small green pepper, chopped

2 garlic cloves, crushed

400 g/14 oz can chopped tomatoes, drained

120 ml/4 fl oz dry red wine

2 tbsp Worcestershire sauce

50 g/2 oz light brown sugar

2 tbsp Dijon mustard

2 tsp celery seeds

salt and freshly ground black pepper, to taste

12 ciabatta rolls, lightly toasted

Cook the beef, onions, pepper and garlic over medium heat in a large frying pan until the beef is browned, crumbling it with a fork. Transfer to the slow cooker. Add the remaining ingredients, except the salt, pepper and rolls. Cover and cook on High for 2–3 hours. Season to taste with salt and pepper. Serve in rolls.

Chicken Burger Buns

Chicken is cooked in a tangy sauce (which contains a surprise ingredient) until meltingly tender and then shredded before it is used to fill burger buns.

Serves 8

450 g/1 lb skinless chicken breast fillets, quartered
350 ml/12 fl oz cola
250 ml/8 fl oz tomato ketchup
75 ml/2½ fl oz yellow mustard
50 g/2 oz light brown sugar
1 onion, chopped
1 garlic clove, crushed
2 tbsp cornflour
50 ml/2 fl oz water
salt and freshly ground black pepper, to taste
8 burger buns

Combine all the ingredients, except the cornflour, water, salt, pepper and buns, in the slow cooker. Cover and cook on Low for 6–8 hours. Turn the heat to High and cook for 10 minutes. Stir in the combined cornflour and water, stirring for 2–3 minutes. Stir to shred the chicken. Season to taste with salt and pepper. Serve in buns.

Punchy Pork Rolls

Sweet and tender pork is shredded and then added to a bun and topped with a garlicky White Barbecue Sauce.

Serves 12

900 g/2 lb boneless pork loin
Brown Sugar Rub (see below)
120 ml/4 fl oz chicken stock
12 small rolls or scones
White Barbecue Sauce (see below)

Rub the pork loin with Brown Sugar Rub. Put in the slow cooker with the stock. Cover and cook on Low for 6–8 hours. Remove the pork and shred. Reserve the cooking liquid for soup or another use. Spoon the meat on to the bottom halves of the rolls and top with White Barbecue Sauce and the roll tops.

Brown Sugar Rub

You could use ground cinnamon if you don't have cumin.

Serves 12

50 g/2 oz light brown sugar

1 tsp garlic powder

½ tsp ground cumin

½ tsp salt

½ tsp pepper

Mix all the ingredients.

White Barbecue Sauce

The horseradish provides an exciting tartness but you can omit it if you're not a fan.

Serves 12

375 ml/13 fl oz mayonnaise

50 ml/2 fl oz cider vinegar

1 tbsp sugar

1 garlic clove, crushed

2 tsp horseradish

1–2 tbsp lemon juice

Mix all the ingredients, adding the lemon juice to taste.

Curry Spice Rub

This rub will keep for weeks in an airtight jar.

1½ tsp curry powder

1½ tsp paprika

¾ tsp ground cinnamon

¾ tsp garlic powder

¾ tsp salt

½ tsp freshly grated nutmeg

½ tsp ground ginger

Combine all the ingredients.

Pork and Chutney Sandwiches

Rub a curry mix into pork before roasting, then serve sliced in granary bread with chutney. You can make your own Mango Chutney, if you like.

Serves 12

900 g/2 lb boneless pork loin
Curry Spice Rub (see below)
120 ml/4 fl oz chicken stock
48 slices granary, ciabatta or sourdough bread
500 g/18 oz mango chutney

Rub the pork loin with Curry Spice Rub. Insert a meat thermometer in the centre of the roast so that the tip is in the centre of the meat. Put the pork in the slow cooker and add the stock. Cover and cook on Low until the meat thermometer registers 71ºC, about 3 hours. Remove the pork to a cutting board and leave to stand, loosely covered with foil, 10 minutes. Reserve the stock for soup or another use. Slice the pork and make sandwiches, spooning about 2 tbsp of chutney into each.

Beef and Provolone Sandwich

Tender beef cooked in wine, then sliced and served in a crusty roll with Provolone makes a fun change. Put the stock in a bowl for dipping.

Serves 12

1.5 kg/3 lb braising steak, in a piece
freshly ground black pepper, to taste
450 ml/¾ pint beef stock
250 ml/8 fl oz dry red wine
1 packet onion soup mix
1 garlic clove, crushed
12 crusty rolls
175 g/6 oz sliced Provolone cheese

Sprinkle the steak lightly with pepper and put in the slow cooker. Add the remaining ingredients, except the rolls and cheese. Cover and cook on Low for 6–8 hours. Remove the steak and slice thinly. Serve the beef on crusty rolls with Provolone cheese slices. Offer the stock for dipping.

Mozzarella Steak Rolls

Sliced steak cooked with onions and peppers is served in a crusty roll with a cheese topping.

Serves 6–8

450 g/1 lb rump steak, thinly sliced

2 onions, thinly sliced

1 green pepper, thinly sliced

250 ml/8 fl oz beef stock

1 garlic clove, crushed

1 tbsp Worcestershire sauce

salt and freshly ground black pepper, to taste

6–8 crusty rolls

175–225 g/6–8 oz Mozzarella cheese, grated

Combine all the ingredients, except the salt, pepper, rolls and cheese, in the slow cooker. Cover and cook on Low for 6–8 hours. Season to taste with salt and pepper. Top the rolls with the meat and vegetable mixture. Sprinkle with cheese. If you like, grill until the cheese has melted, 3–4 minutes.

Hot Focaccia with Salami and Ham

Piquant Olive Relish gives this meat and cheese sandwich plenty of flavour. Make sure the size of the loaf will fit into your slow cooker.

Serves 6

Olive Relish (see below)
1 round focaccia or sourdough loaf (about 20 cm/8 in diameter), halved
100 g/4 oz thinly sliced Italian salami
100 g/4 oz smoked ham, sliced
100 g/4 oz Provolone or Fontina cheese, sliced

Spread half the Olive Relish on the bottom half of the bread. Top with salami, ham and cheese, the remaining Olive Relish and the top of the bread. Press the sandwich together firmly and wrap securely in foil. Line the base of the slow cooker with a large piece of foil. Put the sandwich in the slow cooker. Cover and cook on Low for 2 hours. Cut into wedges to serve.

Olive Relish

Omit the anchovy fillet if you want to make a vegetarian version.

Serves 6

75 g/3 oz pitted black olives, chopped

75 g/3 oz pitted green olives, chopped

90 g/3½ oz tomatoes, chopped

15 g/½ oz fresh parsley, chopped

50 ml/2 fl oz olive oil

1 anchovy fillet, mashed (optional)

juice of ½ lemon

freshly ground black pepper, to taste

Mix all the ingredients, except the pepper. Season to taste with pepper.

Bratwurst Buns with Peppers and Onions

Cook the sausages in beer with peppers, onions and mushrooms, then serve in buns with the savoury vegetables heaped on top. The sausages can be briefly browned in a frying pan or under the grill before serving, if you like.

Serves 6–8

6–8 fresh bratwurst sausages, about 700 g/1½ lb

2–3 x 350 ml/12 fl oz bottles beer

2 onions, chopped

1 red pepper, sliced

1 green pepper, sliced

225 g/8 oz small chestnut mushrooms, sliced

2 garlic cloves, crushed

salt and freshly ground black pepper, to taste

6–8 hot dog buns or soft rolls

Combine all the ingredients, except the salt, pepper and buns, in the slow cooker. Cover and cook on Low for 6–8 hours. Season with salt and pepper. Serve the sausages in buns with the vegetable mixture spooned over.

Polish Sausage and Sauerkraut Rolls

A lovely mixture with typical Polish flavourings.

Serves 4–6

4–6 lean Polish sausages, about 450 g/1 lb

225–350 g/8–12 oz sauerkraut, drained and rinsed

1 onion, thinly sliced

1 small tart eating apple, peeled and thinly sliced

1 tsp fennel seeds

1 tsp caraway seeds

120 ml/4 fl oz chicken stock

freshly ground black pepper, to taste

4–6 hot dog buns or rolls

wholegrain mustard

Put the sausages in the slow cooker. Top with the combined remaining ingredients, except the pepper, buns and mustard. Cover and cook on Low for 6–8 hours. Season to taste with pepper. Serve the sausages and sauerkraut in the buns with mustard.

Italian Beef Rolls

Simple to throw together and tastily cooked to savoury goodness.

Serves 12

1 boneless beef joint such as rump, about 1.5 kg/3 lb

750 ml/1¼ pints beef stock

4 tbsp dried Italian herb seasoning

1 bay leaf

1 tsp freshly ground black pepper

12 buns or ciabatta rolls

Combine all the ingredients, except the buns, in the slow cooker. Cover and cook on Low for 10–12 hours. Remove the meat and shred. Return to the slow cooker. Serve the meat and juices in the buns or rolls.

Aubergine Meatballs with Harlequin Sauce

Granary rolls are filled with Italian-style beef and aubergine meatballs cooked with peppers in a pasta sauce.

Serves 6

Aubergine Meatballs

2 red peppers, sliced

2 green peppers, sliced

450 g/1 lb ready-made pasta sauce, hot

6 large granary or white rolls, lightly toasted on the cut side

Make the Aubergine Meatballs, shaping into 24. Combine the Aubergine Meatballs, peppers and pasta sauce in the slow cooker, covering the meatballs with sauce. Cover and cook on Low for 6–8 hours. Serve in the rolls.

Turkey Pitta Breads

Fill pittas with this zesty mix of turkey with olives, mushrooms and tomatoes.

Serves 8–12

450 g/1 lb boneless, skinless turkey breast or thighs, cubed (5 cm/2 in)

400 g/14 oz can chopped tomatoes

175 g/6 oz ready-made tomato sauce

225 g/8 oz mushrooms, sliced

1 onion, chopped

75 g/3 oz pitted green olives, sliced

1 mild chilli, seeded and sliced

1 tbsp prepared mustard

1 tsp dried oregano

salt and freshly ground black pepper, to taste

4–8 large pitta breads, halved

Combine all the ingredients, except the salt, pepper and pitta breads, in the slow cooker. Cover and cook on Low for 6–8 hours. Season to taste with salt and pepper. Stir to shred the turkey. Serve in pitta halves.

Greek Pitta Breads

A minted cucumber and yoghurt sauce plus crumbled Feta cheese makes a perfect topping for herby lamb meatballs. Minced beef, instead of lamb, for the meatballs would also work well.

Serves 4

450 g/1 lb lean minced lamb
40 g/1½ oz fresh breadcrumbs
1 egg
½ onion, finely chopped
1 tsp dried oregano
1 tsp dried mint
¾ tsp salt
½ tsp pepper
175 ml/6 fl oz chicken stock
2 pitta breads, halved
Cucumber and Yogurt Sauce (see below)
50 g/2 oz Feta cheese, crumbled

Combine the lamb, breadcrumbs, egg, onion, oregano, mint, salt and pepper. Shape into 16 meatballs. Put in the slow cooker with the stock. Cover and cook on Low for 4 hours. Drain and discard the juices, or save for another use. Spoon four meatballs into each pitta half. Top the meatballs in each pitta with 2 tbsp Cucumber and Yogurt sauce and a quarter of the Feta cheese.

Cucumber and Yogurt Sauce

A refreshing sauce that goes well with many Greek and Indian

dishes.

Serves 4

50 ml/2 fl oz yoghurt

50 g/2 oz cucumber, seeded and finely chopped

1 tsp dried mint

Mix all the ingredients.

Moo Shu Wraps

Enjoy the traditional flavours of Chinese spiced pork in a tortilla wrap.

Serves 6

450 g/1 lb pork tenderloin

2 tsp Chinese five-spice powder

2 garlic cloves, crushed

120 ml/4 fl oz plum sauce

50 ml/2 fl oz water

1 tbsp soy sauce

2 cm/¾ in piece fresh root ginger, finely grated

40 g/1½ oz bamboo shoots, cut into thin strips

salt and freshly ground black pepper, to taste

6 x 15 cm/6 in flour tortillas, warmed

120–175 ml/4–6 fl oz hoisin sauce

6 small spring onions

Rub the pork with the Chinese five-spice powder and garlic. Leave to stand for 30 minutes. Put the pork in the slow cooker. Add the combined plum sauce, water, soy sauce and ginger. Cover and cook on Low until the pork is very tender, about 3 hours. Remove the pork and shred with two forks. Return to the slow cooker. Add the bamboo shoots. Cover and cook on Low for 30 minutes. Season to taste with salt and pepper. Spread each tortilla with 1 tbsp hoisin sauce and lay a spring onion in the centre. Divide the pork mixture between the tortillas and roll up.

Picadillo Tortillas

The tenderest cut of pork is cooked with spices and flavourings, then mixed with raisins and almonds to make a superb filling for tortillas, topped with avocado and tomato. They make ideal party food.

Serves 6

350 g/12 oz pork tenderloin

50 ml/2 fl oz water

2 spring onions, thinly sliced

1 garlic clove, crushed,

1 tsp finely chopped jalapeño or other medium-hot chilli, finely chopped

1 tsp ground cinnamon

¼ tsp dried oregano

1–2 tsp cider vinegar

40 g/1½ oz raisins

25 g/1 oz flaked almonds

salt and freshly ground black pepper, to taste

6 x 15 cm/6 in flour tortillas, warmed

150 g/5 oz tomato, chopped

1 avocado, chopped

fresh coriander sprigs, to garnish

salsa, to serve

Combine the pork, water, spring onions, garlic, chilli, cinnamon, oregano and vinegar in the slow cooker. Cover and cook on Low for 3 hours. Remove the pork and shred with 2 forks. Return to the slow cooker. Add the raisins and almonds. Cover and cook on Low for 1 hour. Season to taste with salt and pepper. Divide the pork mixture between the tortillas. Sprinkle with 1 tbsp each of tomato and avocado, and several sprigs of coriander. Roll up and serve with salsa.

Ham, Cheese and Pesto Melts

Serves 4

2–4 tbsp pesto

4 small soft or crusty rolls, halved

100 g/4 oz thinly sliced ham

50 g/2 oz thinly sliced Provolone cheese

Spread the pesto on the bottom halves of the rolls. Top with ham, cheese and the roll tops. Wrap each roll in foil. Put in the slow cooker. Cover and cook on Low for 2 hours. Serve warm.

Turkey Cranberry Melts

Serves 4

50 g/2 oz soft cheese, at room temperature

1 tbsp chopped pecan nuts or walnuts

4 small rolls, halved

100 g/4 oz thinly sliced turkey

4 tbsp cranberry sauce

Spread the combined soft cheese and nuts on the bottom halves of the rolls. Top with the turkey, cranberry sauce and roll tops. Wrap each roll in foil. Put in the slow cooker. Cover and cook on Low for 2 hours. Serve warm.

Goats' Cheese and Salami Melts

Serves 4

50 g/2 oz goats' cheese, at room temperature

50 g/2 oz soft cheese, at room temperature

4 small buns or crusty rolls

2–4 tbsp sun-dried tomato pesto

2–75 g/3 oz thinly sliced salami

Spread the combined goats' and soft cheese on the bottom halves of the buns. Top with the pesto, salami and bun tops. Wrap each bun in foil. Put in the slow cooker. Cover and cook on Low for 2 hours. Serve warm.

Reuben Melts

Serves 4

2–4 tbsp thousand island salad dressing

4 small rye rolls, halved

100 g/4 oz thinly sliced deli-cooked salt beef

4–6 tbsp well-drained sauerkraut

50 g/2 oz thinly sliced Emmental or Gruyère cheese

Spread the salad dressing on the bottom halves of the rolls. Top with the beef, sauerkraut, cheese and roll tops. Wrap each roll in foil. Put in the slow cooker. Cover and cook on Low for 2 hours. Serve warm.

Cucumber Cheese Melts

Serves 4

50 g/2 oz soft cheese, at room temperature

1 tbsp crumbled blue cheese

4 small multigrain rolls, halved

8 thin cucumber slices

2 tbsp apricot jam

Spread the combined soft cheese and blue cheese on the bottom halves of the rolls. Top with the cucumber slices, jam and roll tops. Wrap each roll in foil. Put in the slow cooker. Cover and cook on Low for 2 hours. Serve warm.

Blue Cheese and Pear Melts

Serves 4

50 g/2 oz Cheshire cheese, thinly sliced

4 small soft white or wholemeal rolls

75 g/3 oz orange marmalade

½ small pear, thinly sliced

2 tbsp crumbled blue cheese

Put the Cheshire cheese on the bottom halves of the rolls. Top with the marmalade, pear, blue cheese and roll tops. Wrap each sandwich in foil. Put in the slow cooker. Cover and cook on Low for 2 hours. Serve warm.

Cream Cheese Frosting

Spread this frosting on the cake and, if you like, decorate the top with walnut halves.

makes 300 g/11 oz

50 g/2 oz soft cheese, at room temperature

1 tbsp butter or margarine, at room temperature

½ tsp vanilla essence

250 g/9 oz icing sugar

milk

Beat the cheese, butter or margarine and vanilla essence in a medium bowl until smooth. Beat in the icing sugar and enough milk to make thick topping consistency.

Chocolate Frosting

Ideal for filling and topping sponge cakes.

makes 150 g/5 oz

130 g/4½ oz icing sugar

2 tbsp cocoa powder

½ tsp vanilla essence

milk

Mix the icing sugar, cocoa, vanilla essence and enough milk to make a topping consistency.

Sweet Topping

The butter or margarine needs to be cold, not at room temperature.

Makes enough to fill one cake

20 g/¾ oz cold butter or margarine

2 tbsp flour

2 tbsp sugar

Cut the butter or margarine into the combined flour and sugar until crumbly.

Lemony Carrot Cake with Cream Cheese Frosting

A carrot cake with raisins and walnuts and the zing of lemon.

Serves 12

175 g/6 oz butter or margarine, at room temperature

175 g/6 oz light brown sugar

3 eggs

2 carrots, grated

50 g/2 oz raisins

40 g/1½ oz walnuts, coarsely chopped

grated zest of 1 lemon

175 g/6 oz self-raising flour, plus extra for dusting

1 tsp baking powder

¼ tsp salt

oil, for greasing

Cream Cheese Frosting (see above)

Beat the butter or margarine and sugar in a large bowl until fluffy. Beat in the eggs a little at a time, beating well. Mix in the carrots, raisins, walnuts and lemon zest. Fold in the combined flour, baking powder and salt. Pour into a greased and floured 18 cm/7 in springform cake tin. Put on a rack in a 5.5 litre/9½ pint slow cooker. Cover and cook on High until a cocktail stick inserted into the centre of the cake comes out clean, about 3½ hours. Cool in the tin on a wire rack for 10 minutes. Remove from the tin and allow to cool completely. Spread with Cream Cheese Frosting.

Pumpkin Ginger Cake Rounds with Warm Rum Sauce

Large cans make handy cake tins for baking in the slow cooker. Serve these spiced cakes for dessert, sliced into rounds and accompanied with a warm rum sauce.

makes 2 Cakes, each serves 4–6

100 g/4 oz pumpkin, cooked and mashed

100 g/4 oz light brown sugar

50 g/2 oz butter or margarine, at room temperature

75 g/3 oz golden syrup

1 egg

175 g/6 oz plain flour, plus extra for dusting

½ tsp baking powder

½ tsp bicarbonate of soda

½ tsp ground allspice

½ tsp ground cloves

½ tsp ground ginger

oil, for greasing

Warm Rum Sauce (see below)

Combine the pumpkin, sugar, butter or margarine, syrup and egg in a large mixer bowl. Beat vigorously until well blended. Mix in the combined flour, baking powder, bicarbonate of soda, allspice, cloves and ginger, blending gently until moistened.

Pour the batter into a two greased and floured 450 g/1 lb tins. Stand the tins in the slow cooker. Cover and cook on High until a wooden skewer inserted into the cakes comes out clean, about 2½ hours. Stand the tins on a wire rack to cool for 10 minutes. Loosen the sides of the cakes by gently rolling the tins on the worktop, or remove the bottom ends of the tins and push the cakes through. Slice and serve with Warm Rum Sauce.

Warm Rum Sauce

This goes well with any spicy or fruity cake.

Serves 8–12

50 g/2 oz caster sugar

1 tbsp cornflour

300 ml/½ pint semi-skimmed milk

2 tbsp rum or ½ tsp rum essence

25 g/1 oz butter or margarine

½ tsp vanilla essence

a pinch of freshly grated nutmeg

Mix the sugar and cornflour in a small pan. Whisk in the milk and rum or rum essence. Whisk over medium heat until the mixture boils and thickens, 1–2 minutes. Remove from the heat. Stir in the butter or margarine, vanilla essence and nutmeg. Serve warm.

Vanilla Frosting

If you want to boost the vanilla flavour, add a teaspoonful of vanilla

sugar.

makes 200 g/7 oz

175 g/6 oz icing sugar
1 tsp vanilla essence
6–8 tsp milk

Mix the icing sugar and vanilla essence, adding enough milk to make a thick topping consistency.

Buttercream Frosting

A good topping and filling for sponge cakes.

makes 450 g/1 lb

425 g/15 oz icing sugar

1 tbsp butter or margarine, at room temperature

½ tsp vanilla essence

1–2 tbsp milk

Mix the icing sugar, butter or margarine, vanilla essence and enough milk to make a spreading consistency.

Apple Cake with Vanilla Frosting

Porridge oats add to the homely goodness of this dessert. Serve warm with ice-cream or frozen yoghurt.

Serves 12

100 g/4 oz butter or margarine, at room temperature

175 g/6 oz light brown sugar

1 egg

175 ml/6 fl oz ready-made apple sauce

1 tsp vanilla essence

100 g/4 oz plain flour, plus extra for dusting

50 g/2 oz wholemeal flour

50 g/2 oz porridge oats

2 tsp baking powder

½ tsp salt

½ tsp ground cinnamon

¼ tsp bicarbonate of soda

¼ tsp ground cloves

oil, for greasing

Vanilla Frosting (see above)

Beat the butter or margarine and sugar in a large bowl until blended. Beat in the egg, apple sauce and vanilla essence. Mix in the combined remaining ingredients, except the Vanilla Frosting, stirring until well blended.

Pour the batter into a greased and floured 1.5 litre/2½ pint fluted cake tin. Put the tin on a rack in a 5.5 litre/9½ pint slow cooker. Cover and cook on High until a cocktail stick inserted into the centre of the cake comes out clean, 2½–3 hours. Cool in the tin on a wire rack for 10 minutes. Invert on to the rack and allow to cool completely. Spread with Vanilla Frosting.

Red Velvet Cake

Also known as Waldorf Astoria Cake, this colourful red dessert is reputed to trace its origins to the famed New York hotel. Bizarre though it seems, it really does contain a whole bottle of food colouring.

Serves 8

175 g/6 oz caster sugar

3 tbsp white vegetable fat

1 egg

1 tsp vanilla essence

25 g/1 oz red food colouring

100 g/4 oz cocoa powder

130 g/4½ oz plain flour, plus extra for dusting

1 tsp bicarbonate of soda

½ tsp salt

120 ml/4 fl oz buttermilk

1½ tsp white distilled vinegar

oil, for greasing

Buttercream Frosting

Beat the sugar and fat in a large bowl until well blended. Add the egg and vanilla essence, blending well. Beat in the food colouring and cocoa until well blended. Mix in the combined flour, bicarbonate of soda and salt alternately with the combined buttermilk and vinegar, beginning and ending with the dry ingredients.

Pour the batter into a greased and floured 1 litre/1¾ pint soufflé dish. Put on a rack in a 5.5 litre/9½ pint slow cooker. Cover and cook on High until a cocktail stick inserted into the centre of the cake comes out clean, 2–2¾ hours. Remove to a wire rack and cool in the tin for 10 minutes. Invert on to the rack and allow to cool completely. Spread with Buttercream Frosting.

Chocolate Chip Peanut Butter Cake

Chocolate and peanut butter – a comfort food combination that can't be beaten. Serve as a dessert with chocolate sauce, if you like.

Serves 8

65 g/2½ oz butter or margarine, at room temperature

65 g/2½ oz caster sugar

65 g/2½ oz light brown sugar

2 eggs

100 g/4 oz crunchy peanut butter

120 ml/4 fl oz soured cream

190 g/6½ oz self-raising flour, plus extra for dusting

¼ tsp salt

50 g/2 oz plain chocolate chips

oil, for greasing

chocolate sauce (optional)

Beat the butter or margarine and sugars in a bowl until fluffy. Beat in the eggs, blending well. Mix in the peanut butter and soured cream. Mix in the flour, salt and chocolate chips.

Pour the batter into a greased and floured 1.5 litre/2½ pint fluted cake tin. Put on a rack in a 5.5 litre/9½ pint slow cooker. Cover and cook on High until a cocktail stick inserted into the centre of the cake comes out clean, 2–2½ hours. Cool in the tin on a wire rack for 10 minutes. Invert on to the rack and allow to cool completely. Serve with chocolate sauce.

Chocolate Sauerkraut Cake

Vegetables are often added to cakes to make them beautifully moist. In this cake there are two unusual ingredients for a delicious cake: sauerkraut and beer.

Serves 8

175 g/6 oz caster sugar

50 g/2 oz white vegetable fat

1 egg

1 tsp vanilla essence

25 g/1 oz cocoa powder

130 g/4½ oz plain flour, plus extra for dusting

½ tsp baking powder

½ tsp bicarbonate of soda

¼ tsp salt

120 ml/4 fl oz beer

40 g/1½ oz sauerkraut, rinsed, well-drained and finely chopped

oil, for greasing

Chocolate Frosting

Beat the sugar and fat in a large bowl until blended. Beat in the egg, vanilla essence and cocoa. Mix in the combined flour, baking powder, bicarbonate of soda and salt alternately with the beer, beginning and ending with the dry ingredients. Mix in the sauerkraut.

Pour the batter into a greased and floured 1.5 litre/2½ pint fluted cake tin. Put on a rack in a 5.5 litre/9½ pint slow cooker. Cover and cook on High until a cocktail stick inserted into the centre of the cake comes out clean, 2½–3 hours. Cool in the tin on a wire rack for 10 minutes. Invert on to the rack and allow to cool completely.Spread the Chocolate Frosting over.

Date and Nut Ginger Slices

For a really delicious treat, spread the cake slices with softened cheese and apricot preserve.

makes 2 Cakes, each serves 4–6

100 g/4 oz pumpkin, cooked and mashed

100 g/4 oz light brown sugar

50 g/2 oz butter or margarine, at room temperature

75 g/3 oz golden syrup

1 egg

175 g/6 oz plain flour, plus extra for dusting

½ tsp baking powder

½ tsp bicarbonate of soda

½ tsp ground allspice

½ tsp ground cloves

½ tsp ground ginger

40 g/1½ oz dates, chopped

25 g/1 oz walnuts, chopped

oil, for greasing

Combine the pumpkin, sugar, butter or margarine, syrup and egg in a large mixer bowl. Beat vigorously until well blended. Mix in the combined flour, baking powder, bicarbonate of soda, allspice, cloves and ginger, blending gently until moistened. Stir in the dates and walnuts.

Pour the batter into a two greased and floured 450 g/1 lb tins. Stand the tins in the slow cooker. Cover and cook on High until a wooden skewer inserted into the cakes comes out clean, about 2½ hours. Stand the tins on a wire rack to cool for 10 minutes. Loosen the sides of the cakes by gently rolling the tins on the worktop, or remove the bottom ends of the tins and push the cakes through. Slice and serve.

Gingerbread Cake

Enjoy this moist and perfectly spiced cake with its cream cheese topping.

Serves 12

175 g/6 oz self-raising flour

50 g/2 oz plain flour

1 tsp ground cinnamon

½ tsp ground ginger

¼ tsp ground allspice

¼ tsp salt

100 g/4 oz butter or margarine, at room temperature

225 g/8 oz golden syrup

175 g/6 oz light brown sugar

1 egg, lightly beaten

120 ml/4 fl oz semi-skimmed milk

½ tsp bicarbonate of soda

oil, for greasing

Cream Cheese Frosting

Combine the flours, spices and salt in a large bowl. Combine the butter or margarine, syrup and sugar in a 1 litre/1¾ pint glass measuring jug. Microwave on High until the butter or margarine is melted, about 2 minutes, stirring to blend. Whisk the butter mixture into the flour mixture, blending well. Whisk in the egg. Whisk in the combined milk and bicarbonate of soda until blended.

Pour the batter into a greased and floured 18 cm/7 in springform cake tin. Put on a rack in the slow cooker. Cover and cook on High until a cocktail stick inserted into the centre of the cake comes out clean, about 5 hours. Cool in the tin on a wire rack for 10 minutes. Remove the side of the tin and allow to cool completely. Spread with Cream Cheese Frosting.

Chocolate Courgette Cake

Chocolate cakes can be disappointingly dry in texture, but not when one of the ingredients is courgettes. Top this moist and spicy cake with Chocolate Frosting, if you like.

Serves 8

50 g/2 oz butter or margarine, at room temperature

50 ml/2 fl oz ready-made apple sauce

175 g/6 oz caster sugar

1 egg

50 ml/2 fl oz buttermilk

1 tsp vanilla essence

150 g/5 oz plain flour, plus extra for dusting

2 tbsp cocoa powder

½ tsp bicarbonate of soda

½ tsp baking powder

¼ tsp salt

¼ tsp ground cinnamon

¼ tsp ground cloves

175 g/6 oz courgettes, finely chopped or grated

25 g/1 oz plain chocolate chips

oil, for greasing

icing sugar, to decorate

Beat the butter or margarine, apple sauce and sugar in a large bowl until smooth. Mix in the egg, buttermilk and vanilla essence. Mix in the combined flour, cocoa, bicarbonate of soda, baking powder, salt and spices. Mix in the courgettes and chocolate chips.

Pour the batter into a greased and floured 1.5 litre/2½ pint fluted cake tin. Put the tin on a rack in a 5.5 litre/9½ pint slow cooker. Cover and cook on High until a cocktail stick inserted into the centre of the cake comes out clean, 3–4 hours. Cool in the tin on a wire rack for 10 minutes. Invert the cake on to the rack and allow to cool completely. Sprinkle generously with icing sugar.

Chocolate and Coffee Cake

The flavours of coffee and chocolate were made in heaven! This cake can also be baked in a greased 2.75 litre/4¾ pint slow cooker. Cooking time will be about 2½ hours. Using foil handles will make this cake easier to remove from the slow cooker.

Serves 12

6 tbsp butter or margarine, at room temperature

275 g/10 oz caster sugar

2 eggs

100 g/4 oz plain flour, plus extra for dusting

40 g/1½ oz cocoa powder

½ tsp bicarbonate of soda

¼ tsp baking powder

¼ tsp salt

1–2 tbsp instant or espresso coffee

1–2 tbsp boiling water

75 ml/2½ fl oz soured cream

oil, for greasing

Coffee Frosting

Beat the butter or margarine and sugar in a bowl until fluffy. Beat in the eggs a little at a time, beating well after each addition. Mix in the combined dry ingredients alternately with the combined coffee, boiling water and soured cream, beginning and ending with the dry ingredients. Pour the batter into a greased and floured 1.5 litre/2½ pint fluted cake tin. Put the tin on a rack in a 5.5 litre/ 9½ pint slow cooker. Cover and cook on High until a cocktail stick inserted into the centre of the cake comes out clean, 4–4½ hours. Cool in the tin on a wire rack for 10 minutes. Invert the cake on to the rack and allow to cool completely. Spread the cake with Coffee Frosting.